The secrets of Gut Health Cookbook.

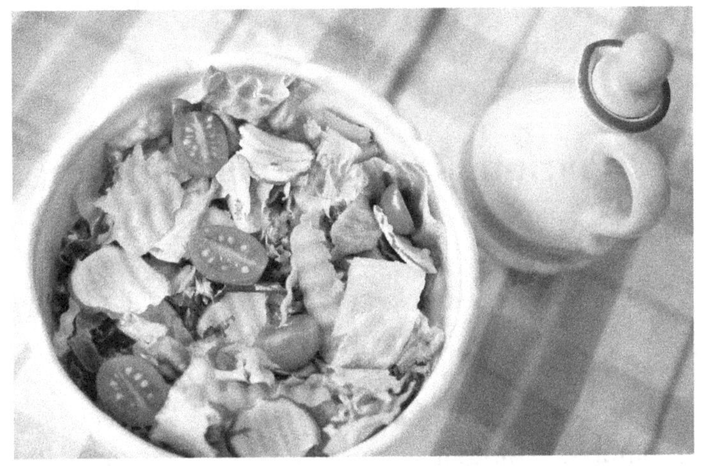

Nourishing Recipes for Gut Bliss

Cameron Brooks

Table of content

Table of content   **3**

INTRODUCTION   **7**

PART ONE   **10**

"The Microbial Symphony: Unraveling the Wonders of Your Gut Ecosystem"   **10**

CHAPTER ONE: **11**

UNDERSTANDING THE WORLD OF OUR GUT MICROBES.   11

1. Diversity and Composition   11

2. Functionality   12

3. Immune System Interaction   12

4. Brain-Gut Axis   12

5. Health Implications   13

6. Impact of Diet   13

7. Antibiotics and Disruptions   13

8. Therapeutic Potential   14

9. Ongoing Research   14

CHAPTER TWO: **15**

EFFECTS OF NOT MAINTAINING PROPER GUT HEALTH   15

CHAPTER THREE: **21**

HEALING YOUR GUT   21

1. Understanding Your Gut Microbiota   21

2. The Gut-Brain Connection   22

3. Probiotics   22

4. Prebiotics 23

5. Fiber 23

6. Healing Foods for Gut Health 24

7. The Impact of Stress on Your Gut 24

8. Hydration 24

9. Identifying and Addressing Food Sensitivities 25

10. Lifestyle Practices for Gut Health 25

DOS AND DON'TS TO MAINTAIN A GOOD GUT HEALTH 26

Dos for Perfect Gut Health: 26

Don'ts for Perfect Gut Health: 28

PART TWO **32**

Beginning With Your New Diet **32**

CHAPTER FOUR **33**

THE 4 WEEK PLAN **33**

The Full Four-Week Plan With Recipes 35

Week 1: Diversify Your Plate 35

Week 2: Embrace Probiotic Foods 47

Week 3: Boost Fiber Intake 61

Week 4: Mindful Eating and Hydration 76

ADDITIONAL TIPS FOR EACH WEEK 90

CHAPTER FIVE **91**

Post Four-Week Plan **91**

Post Four-Week Recipes 92

Week 5: Vibrant Gut Rejuvenation 92

Week 6: Colors of the Garden 102

Week 7: Mediterranean Flavors 110

Week 8: Fusion Fiesta 118

Conclusion **127**

INTRODUCTION

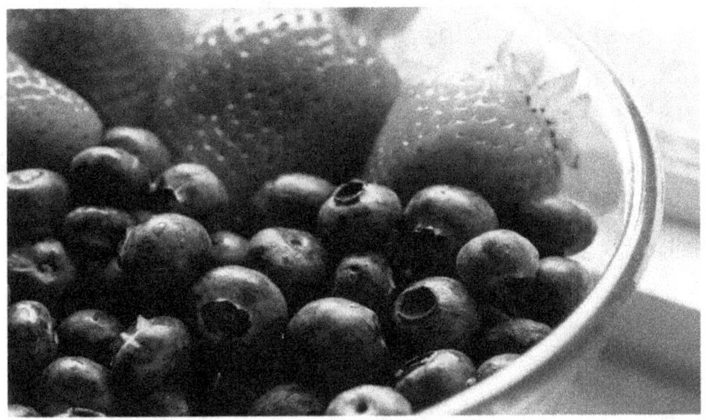

Welcome, culinary explorers, to the vibrant realm of the "Secrets of Gut Health Cookbook," where we unravel the delectable mysteries that lie at the intersection of flavor and well-being. Prepare to embark on a gastronomic adventure that not only tantalizes your taste buds but also nourishes the epicenter of vitality – your gut.

In these pages, we unveil a treasure trove of culinary secrets, carefully curated to empower you with the knowledge and recipes needed to cultivate a thriving gut. Think of it as your passport to a world where delicious meets nutritious, and where every bite contributes to the harmonious symphony of your body's well-being.

Imagine unlocking the culinary alchemy that transforms ordinary meals into a feast for your gut microbiome. From mouthwatering dishes designed to pamper your palate to refreshing elixirs that invigorate from within, this cookbook is your compass for navigating the exciting landscape of gut health.

But it's not just about what's on your plate – it's a journey of discovery. Delve into the fascinating insights shared by nutrition experts, unraveling the intricate dance between food and gut function. Learn the art of creating meals that not only satiate your cravings but also foster a happy, balanced gut environment.

Prepare to be captivated by the diversity of recipes, each a delightful expression of the belief that taking care of your gut should be an indulgent experience. This is more than a cookbook; it's a celebration of the powerful connection between the pleasure of eating and the science of well-being.

So, buckle up for a culinary odyssey that transcends the ordinary, where the kitchen becomes your sanctuary, and each recipe is a carefully crafted potion for a healthier, happier you. The secrets are unveiled, the flavors are calling – welcome to the Secrets of Gut Health Cookbook, your gateway to a world where good food is the ultimate elixir.

Each recipe is a delectable exploration, marrying flavours that ignite the senses with ingredients scientifically selected to promote a harmonious gut environment. From fermented delights to fiber-rich wonders, every dish is a step toward a more balanced and resilient digestive system.

But this cookbook is more than a collection of recipes; it's a holistic approach to wellness. Alongside mouth watering creations, you'll find insights into the science behind gut health, practical tips for mindful eating, and a guide to understanding your body's unique needs.

Join us on this gastronomic adventure, where taste and health converge, unlocking the secrets to a vibrant, thriving gut and a happier, healthier you.

PART ONE

"The Microbial Symphony: Unraveling the Wonders of Your Gut Ecosystem"

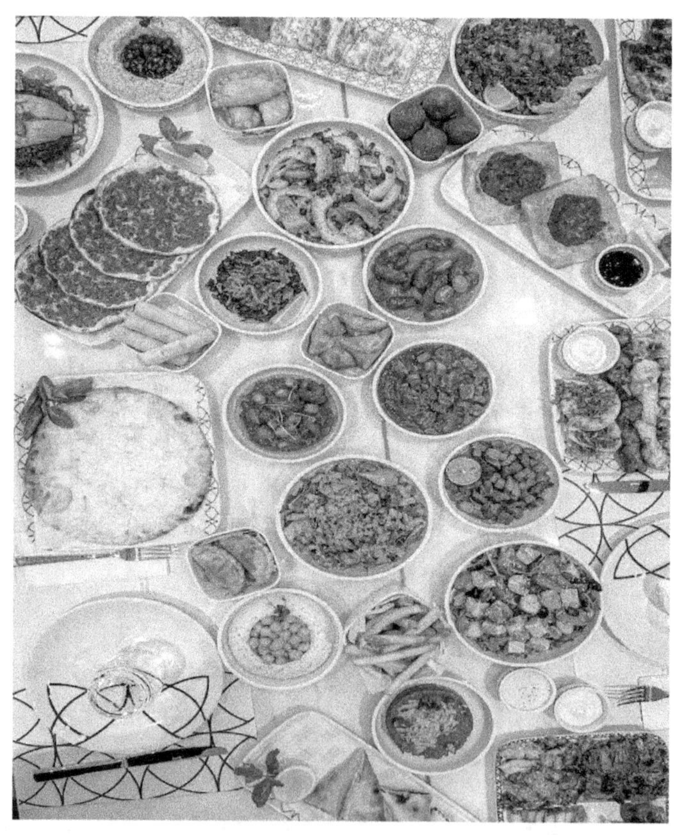

CHAPTER ONE:

UNDERSTANDING THE WORLD OF OUR GUT MICROBES.

The world of our gut microbes, collectively known as the gut microbiota, is a complex ecosystem consisting of trillions of microorganisms, including bacteria, viruses, fungi, and archaea. This intricate community plays a crucial role in maintaining our overall health and well-being.

1. Diversity and Composition

- The gut microbiota is highly diverse, with various species coexisting in a dynamic balance. Factors like diet, genetics, and environment influence its composition.

2. Functionality

- Gut microbes aid in digestion and nutrient absorption, particularly fermenting complex carbohydrates that our bodies cannot digest alone.

- They produce essential vitamins and metabolites, contributing to our overall nutritional status.

3. Immune System Interaction

- The gut microbiota interacts with the immune system, influencing its development and responsiveness.

- A balanced microbiota helps prevent harmful pathogens from colonizing the gut.

4. Brain-Gut Axis

- The bidirectional communication between the gut and the brain, known as the brain-gut axis, involves complex signal pathways. Gut microbes can influence mood, behavior, and cognitive function, contributing to the emerging field of microbiome-brain interactions.

5. Health Implications

- Imbalances in the gut microbiota, known as dysbiosis, have been linked to various health conditions, including inflammatory bowel diseases, obesity, and autoimmune disorders.

- Research shows that these imbalances play a potential role in mental health disorders like depression and anxiety.

6. Impact of Diet

- Dietary choices significantly influence the gut microbiota. A diverse and balanced diet rich in fiber supports microbial diversity and a healthier gut environment.

7. Antibiotics and Disruptions

- Antibiotic use can disrupt the balance of gut microbes, leading to short-term and sometimes long-term changes in the microbiota composition.

- Strategies to restore a healthy microbiota after antibiotic treatment are actively researched.

8. Therapeutic Potential

- Probiotics, prebiotics, and fecal microbiota transplantation (FMT) are areas of exploration for therapeutic interventions to modulate the gut microbiota and address certain health conditions.

9. Ongoing Research

- Scientific understanding of the gut microbiota is continually evolving, with ongoing research exploring its role in diverse aspects of human health, including metabolism, cardiovascular health, and even the development of certain cancers.

In essence, the world within our gut is a fascinating and vital aspect of human biology, with far-reaching implications for our health and the potential for innovative therapeutic interventions.

CHAPTER TWO:

EFFECTS OF NOT MAINTAINING PROPER GUT HEALTH

When gut health is not properly maintained, it can lead to a range of adverse effects on overall well-being. Here's a comprehensive look at what happens when the delicate balance of the gut microbiota is disrupted:

1. Digestive Issues:

   - Imbalance in Gut Flora: Disruptions in the gut microbiota can result in an overgrowth of harmful bacteria, leading to conditions like dysbiosis.

   - Constipation or Diarrhea: Irregularities in bowel movements can occur, ranging from constipation to diarrhea.

2. Nutrient Absorption Impairment:

   - A compromised gut can hinder the absorption of essential nutrients, potentially leading to nutrient deficiencies and related health issues.

3. Weakened Immune System:

   - The gut plays a crucial role in immune system modulation. Poor gut health may compromise immune function, making the body more susceptible to infections and illnesses.

4. Inflammation:

   - Chronic inflammation can arise from an imbalanced gut microbiome, contributing to a variety of health conditions, including inflammatory bowel diseases (IBD) and autoimmune disorders.

5. Weight Management Challenges:

   - An unhealthy gut can be linked to difficulties in weight management. It may contribute to obesity or difficulties in losing weight.

6. Mental Health Implications:

- The gut-brain axis influences mental health. Poor gut health has been associated with conditions like anxiety, depression, and mood disorders.

7. Increased Risk of Chronic Diseases:

   - Conditions such as cardiovascular diseases, diabetes, and certain cancers have been linked to imbalances in gut health.

8. Food Intolerances:

   - A compromised gut lining can lead to increased permeability (leaky gut), potentially causing food particles to enter the bloodstream and triggering immune responses, leading to food intolerances.

9. Skin Issues:

   - Skin conditions like acne, eczema, and psoriasis can be influenced by gut health, as the gut-skin axis plays a role in maintaining skin homeostasis.

10. Fatigue and Low Energy:

   - Poor gut health can contribute to feelings of fatigue and low energy levels, impacting overall vitality.

11. Insulin Resistance:

   - Imbalances in the gut microbiota may contribute to insulin resistance, a precursor to diabetes.

12. Increased Allergic Reactions:

   - A compromised gut can lead to an overactive immune response, potentially increasing the risk of allergic reactions.

13. Difficulty in Healing:

   - Slower recovery from injuries or illnesses may occur due to the weakened immune system and impaired nutrient absorption.

14. Risk of Gastrointestinal Disorders:

- Long-term neglect of gut health may elevate the risk of developing gastrointestinal disorders such as irritable bowel syndrome (IBS), Crohn's disease, or ulcerative colitis.

Maintaining proper gut health through a balanced diet, stress management, and a healthy lifestyle is crucial for overall well-being. If persistent gut issues are experienced, seeking advice from healthcare professionals or registered dietitians is recommended for personalized guidance and intervention.

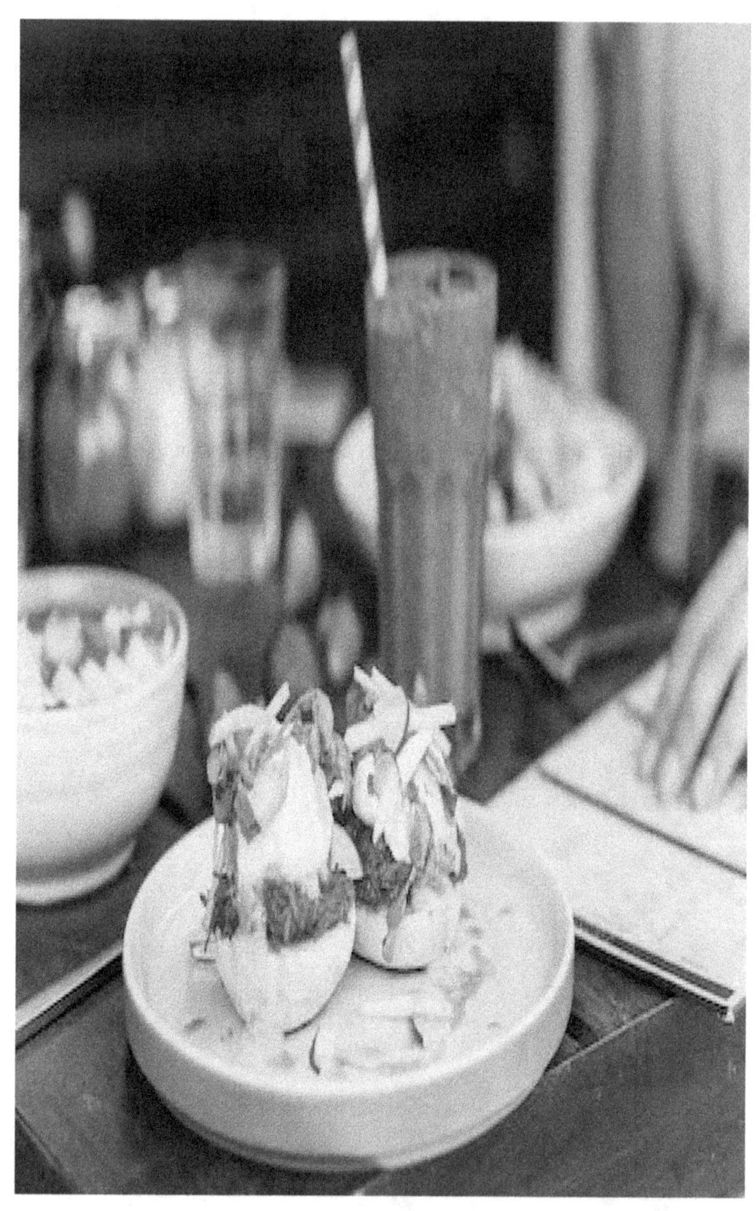

CHAPTER THREE:

HEALING YOUR GUT

A healthy gut is fundamental to overall well-being, impacting digestion, immunity, and even mental health. This comprehensive guide explores various strategies to heal your gut and promote a flourishing microbiome.

Healing your gut involves adopting lifestyle changes and dietary practices that promote a balanced and healthy gut microbiota.

Remember that healing your gut is a gradual process, and individual responses may vary. It's essential to make sustainable lifestyle changes and, if needed, seek guidance from healthcare professionals for a more personalized approach.

1. Understanding Your Gut Microbiota

The gut microbiota comprises trillions of microorganisms residing in your digestive tract. These include bacteria, viruses, fungi, and

archaea, forming a complex ecosystem.
Understanding this intricate world is the first
step towards fostering gut health.

2. The Gut-Brain Connection

Research has unveiled the bidirectional
communication between the gut and the brain,
known as the gut-brain axis. This connection
influences not only digestion but also mood and
mental health.

3. Probiotics

The Beneficial BacteriaProbiotics are live
microorganisms that confer health benefits
when consumed in adequate amounts. They
play a pivotal role in maintaining a balanced gut
microbiota.Incorporating Probiotics into Your
Diet:

Yogurt with live cultures

Kefir

Fermented vegetables (e.g., sauerkraut, kimchi)

Kombucha

4. Prebiotics

Nourishing Your Microbial FriendsPrebiotics are non-digestible fibers that feed the beneficial bacteria in your gut. Including prebiotic-rich foods in your diet promotes a thriving microbiomeFoods High in Prebiotics:

Garlic

Onions

Bananas

5. Fiber

Nature's Broom for Your Gut. Dietary fiber is essential for gut health, aiding in digestion and supporting the growth of beneficial bacteria.

Fiber-Rich Choices:

Whole grains (quinoa, oats)

Legumes (lentils, chickpeas)

Fruits (apples, berries)

Vegetables (broccoli, Brussels sprouts)

6. Healing Foods for Gut Health

Certain foods possess anti-inflammatory and healing properties beneficial for gut health.Include These Healing Foods:

Fatty fish (salmon, mackerel)

Turmeric

Ginger

Leafy greens (kale, spinach)

7. The Impact of Stress on Your Gut

Chronic stress can disrupt the balance of your gut microbiota, emphasizing the importance of stress management for gut health.
Stress-Reducing Activities:

Meditation

Yoga

Regular exercise

8. Hydration

A Key to Gut WellnessAdequate water intake supports the mucosal lining of the intestines, aiding in digestion and nutrient absorption. Stay Hydrated with:

WaterHerbal teas

Infused water with fruits and herbs

9. Identifying and Addressing Food Sensitivities

Unidentified food sensitivities can contribute to gut issues. Identifying and eliminating trigger foods can be crucial for gut healing.Image: Food Sensitivity Testing

Common Food Sensitivity Culprits:

GlutenDairy

Certain FODMAPs (fermentable carbohydrates)

10. Lifestyle Practices for Gut Health

Beyond diet, lifestyle choices profoundly impact gut health. Incorporating these practices contributes to a holistic approach. Healthy Lifestyle Habits:

Adequate sleep

Regular physical activity

Limited alcohol consumption

DOS AND DON'TS TO MAINTAIN A GOOD GUT HEALTH

HERE ARE SOME DOS AND DON'TS TO MAINTAIN A GOOD GUT HEALTH:

Dos for Perfect Gut Health:

1. **Consume a varied Diet:**

   -To encourage a varied gut flora, eat a range of fruits, vegetables, healthy grains, and lean proteins

2. **Include Probiotic-Rich Foods:**

   - Incorporate foods like yogurt, kefir, sauerkraut, kimchi, and kombucha to introduce beneficial bacteria into your gut.

3. **Bone Broth:**

   - Consider incorporating bone broth into your diet. It contains collagen and amino acids that can support gut integrity.

4. **Prioritize Fiber Intake:**

   - Choose fiber-rich foods such as whole grains, legumes, and plenty of fruits and vegetables to support digestive health.

5. **Stay Hydrated:**

   - Drink an adequate amount of water throughout the day to maintain the mucosal lining of the intestines and support digestion.

6. **Manage Stress:**

   - Practice stress-reducing activities like meditation, yoga, or deep breathing to positively impact gut health.

7. **Get Regular Exercise:**

   - Engage in regular physical activity to promote a healthy gut microbiota and overall digestive function.

8. **Adequate Sleep:**

- Ensure you get sufficient and quality sleep, as it contributes to overall well-being, including gut health.

9. Chew Food Thoroughly:

- Chew your food well to aid digestion and make it easier for your gut to absorb nutrients.

10. Include Anti-Inflammatory Foods:

- Consume foods with anti-inflammatory properties, such as fatty fish, turmeric, ginger, and green leafy vegetables.

11. Consider Prebiotics:

Prebiotic-rich foods such as garlic, onions, bananas, and asparagus can help to nourish good gut bacteria

Don'ts for Perfect Gut Health:

1. Avoid Excessive Sugar:

- Limit intake of refined sugars and sugary beverages, as they can disrupt the balance of gut bacteria.

2. Reduce Processed Foods:

- Minimize the consumption of highly processed foods, as they often lack the nutrients necessary for gut health.

3. Limit Artificial Sweeteners:

- Be cautious with artificial sweeteners, as they may negatively impact the gut microbiota.

4. Avoid Overuse of Antibiotics:

- Use antibiotics judiciously and only when prescribed by a healthcare professional to prevent disruptions in gut flora.

5. Don't Skip Meals:

- Avoid skipping meals, as regular eating patterns help maintain a healthy gut environment.

6. **Limit Alcohol Intake:**

   - Consume alcohol in moderation, as excessive alcohol can adversely affect gut health.

7. **Avoid Smoking:**

   - Quit smoking, as it can contribute to gut-related issues and negatively impact overall health.

8. **Minimize Stressful Situations:**

   - Reduce exposure to chronic stressors, as prolonged stress can negatively affect the gut-brain axis.

9. **Avoid Overuse of Antibacterial Products:**

- Limit the use of antibacterial soaps and cleansers, as they may disrupt the natural balance of gut bacteria.

10. **Be Mindful of Food Sensitivities:**

- Identify and manage any food sensitivities or allergies that may contribute to gut issues.

Remember, achieving and maintaining perfect gut health is an ongoing process that involves a combination of healthy dietary and lifestyle choices. Individual responses may vary, so it's important to find a balance that works for your unique needs. If you have specific concerns, consult with a healthcare professional or a registered dietitian for personalized advice.

Always consult with a healthcare professional or a registered dietitian for personalized advice tailored to specific digestive issues.

PART TWO

Beginning With Your New Diet

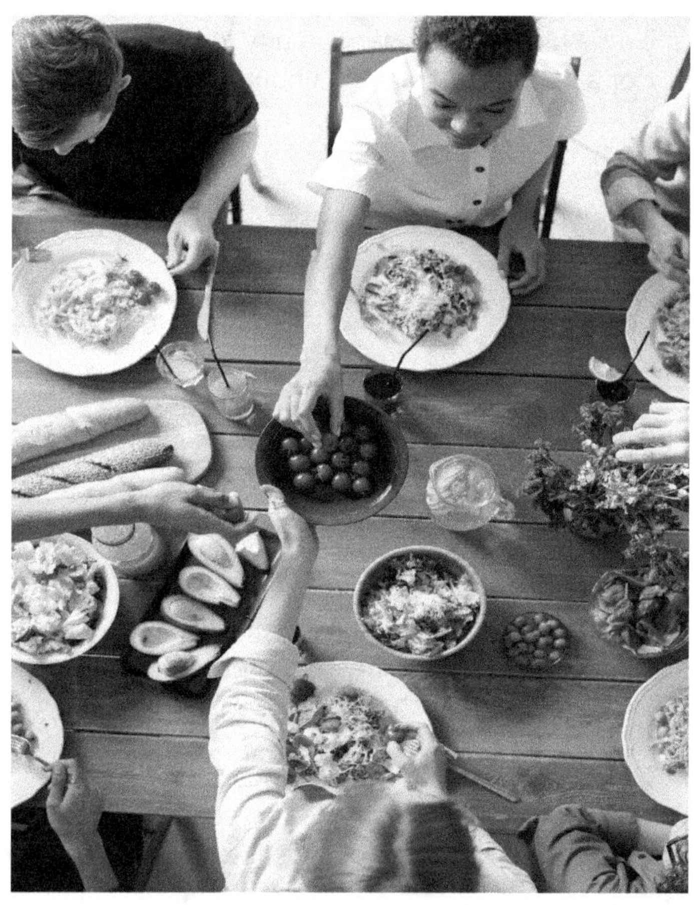

CHAPTER FOUR

THE 4 WEEK PLAN

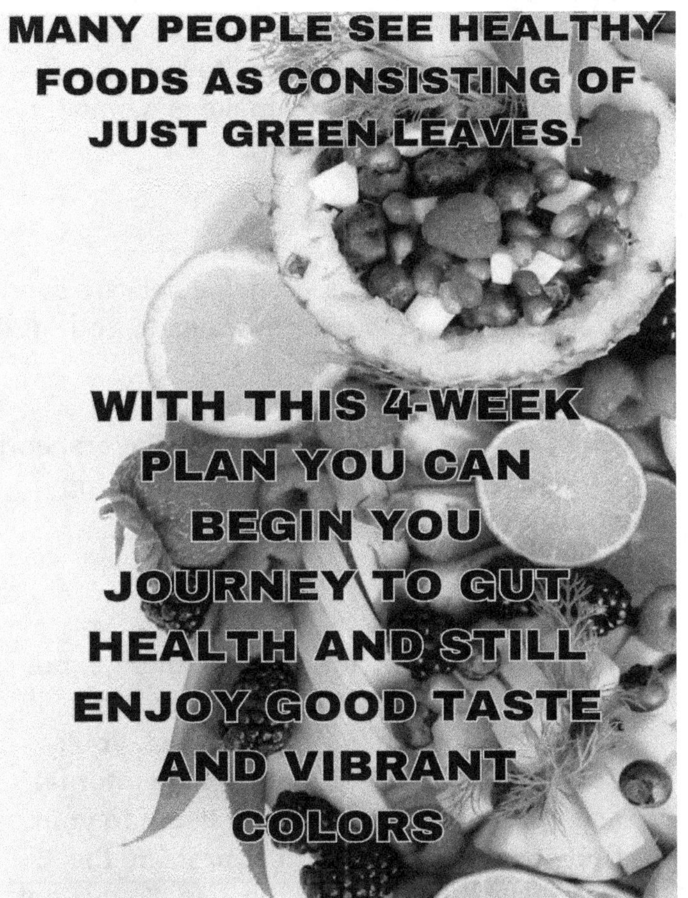

Embarking on this four-week journey to prioritize your gut health is a powerful decision! Remember, it's not just about what you're giving up; it's about embracing a healthier, more nourishing lifestyle. Each nutrient-rich choice you make is a small victory for your well-being.

As you start this eating plan, celebrate every step forward, no matter how small. Your gut will thank you for the wholesome, gut-friendly foods you'll be enjoying. Embrace the process, savor the flavors, and trust that your commitment to nurturing your gut will yield positive results.

There might be moments of challenge, but view them as opportunities for growth. You're not just changing your diet; you're cultivating a resilient and thriving internal ecosystem. Stay consistent, listen to your body, and don't forget to appreciate the positive changes along the way. You've got this!

The Full Four-Week Plan With Recipes

Week 1: Diversify Your Plate

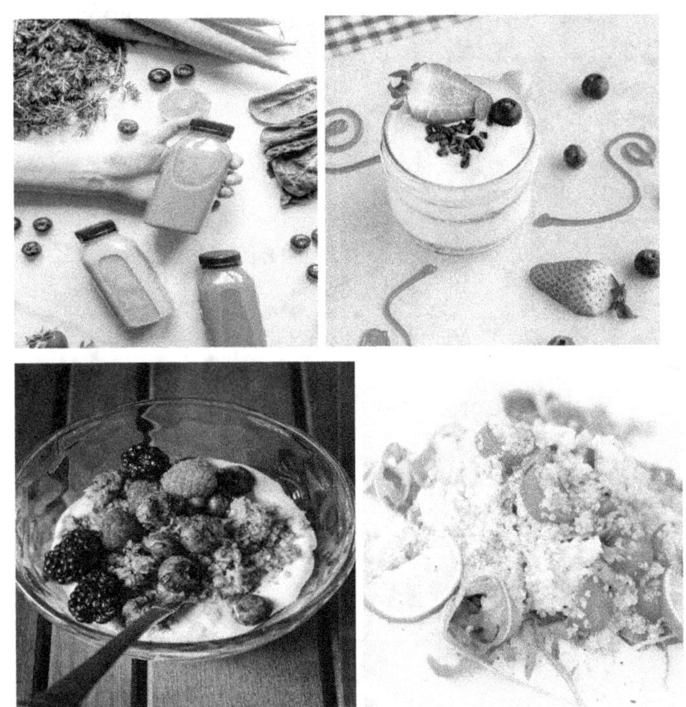

Day 1-7:

- Breakfast:

- Greek yoghurt parfait topped with chia seeds and a mixture of fruit.

Ingredients:

- 1 cup Greek yogurt

- 2 tablespoons honey

- 1 teaspoon vanilla extract

- 2 tablespoons chia seeds

- 1 cup mixed berries (strawberries, blueberries, raspberries)

- 1 ripe mango, diced

- 1/4 cup granola

Instructions:

1. In a bowl, mix Greek yogurt with honey and vanilla extract until well combined.

2. Stir in chia seeds and let the mixture sit for at least 30 minutes or refrigerate overnight for a thicker consistency.

3. In serving glasses or bowls, start layering the parfait. Begin with a spoonful of the Greek yogurt and chia seed mixture.

4. Add a layer of mixed berries, distributing them evenly.

5. Follow with a layer of diced mango for a tropical twist.

6. Repeat the layers until you reach the top of the glass, finishing with a dollop of the Greek yogurt mixture.

7. Sprinkle granola on top for added crunch and texture.

8. Optional: Drizzle a bit of honey over the parfait for extra sweetness.

9. Serve immediately and enjoy a delightful, nutritious Greek yogurt parfait with the

goodness of chia seeds and a burst of fresh fruit flavors.

- **Lunch:**

  - Quinoa salad with colorful vegetables, chickpeas, and a lemon-tahini dressing.

Ingredients:

For the Salad:

- 1 cup quinoa, rinsed and cooked according to package instructions

- 1 can (15 oz) chickpeas, drained and rinsed

- 1 cup cherry tomatoes, halved

- 1 cucumber, diced

- 1 red bell pepper, diced

- 1/2 red onion, finely chopped

- 1/2 cup Kalamata olives, sliced

- 1/4 cup fresh parsley, chopped

For the Lemon-Tahini Dressing:

- 1/4 cup tahini

- 3 tablespoons olive oil

- Zest and juice of 1 lemon

- 2 cloves garlic, minced

- 1 tablespoon honey

- Salt and pepper to taste

Instructions:

1. Cook quinoa according to package instructions and let it cool.

2. In a large bowl, combine the cooked quinoa, chickpeas, cherry tomatoes, cucumber, red bell pepper, red onion, olives, and parsley.

3. In a separate bowl, whisk together tahini, olive oil, lemon zest, lemon juice, minced garlic, honey, salt, and pepper. Adjust the seasoning to your liking.

4. Pour the lemon-tahini dressing over the quinoa and vegetable mIxture. Toss well to ensure everything is evenly coated.

5. Allow the salad to marinate in the dressing for at least 15 minutes to let the flavors meld.

6. Before serving, give the salad a final toss and garnish with additional parsley if desired.

7. Serve chilled or at room temperature as a refreshing and nutritious meal on its own or as a side dish.

Enjoy this vibrant quinoa salad packed with colorful veggies, protein-rich chickpeas, and a zesty lemon-tahini dressing!

- **Dinner:**

  - Baked salmon served with steamed broccoli and roasted sweet potatoes.

Ingredients:

For Baked Salmon:

- 4 salmon fillets

- 2 tablespoons olive oil

- 2 tablespoons lemon juice

- 2 cloves garlic, minced

- 1 teaspoon dried dill

- Salt and pepper to taste

For Roasted Sweet Potatoes:

- 3 medium sweet potatoes, peeled and diced

- 2 tablespoons olive oil

- 1 teaspoon smoked paprika

- Salt and pepper to taste

For Steamed Broccoli:

- 1 lb broccoli florets

- Lemon wedges for serving

Instructions:

Baked Salmon:

1. Preheat the oven to 375°F (190°C).

2. Place salmon fillets on a parchment-lined baking sheet.

3. In a small bowl, mix olive oil, lemon juice, minced garlic, dried dill, salt, and pepper.

4. Brush the salmon fillets with the mixture, ensuring they are well-coated.

5. Bake for 12-15 minutes or until the salmon is cooked through and flakes easily with a fork.

Roasted Sweet Potatoes:

1. Preheat the oven to 400°F (200°C).

2. In a large bowl, toss sweet potato cubesSpread the potatoes on a baking sheet in a single layer. with olive oil, smoked paprika, salt, and pepper.

3. Place the sweet potatoes in a single layer on a baking pan.

4. Roast for 25-30 minutes or until the sweet potatoes are tender and slightly crispy.

Steamed Broccoli:

1. Steam broccoli florets until they are bright green and tender-crisp, about 5-7 minutes.

Assemble:

1. Arrange the baked salmon fillets on plates.

2. Serve alongside steamed broccoli and roasted sweet potatoes.

3. Garnish with additional lemon wedges for a burst of freshness.

4. Optional: Drizzle any remaining lemon-garlic-dill mixture from the salmon over the dish for extra flavor.

Enjoy this wholesome and delicious meal of baked salmon, steamed broccoli, and roasted sweet potatoes!

Snacks:

 - Fresh fruit (e.g., apple slices with almond butter) and a small handful of mixed nuts.

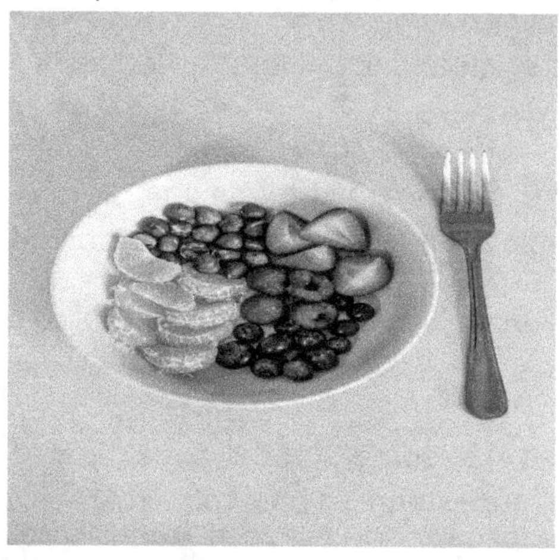

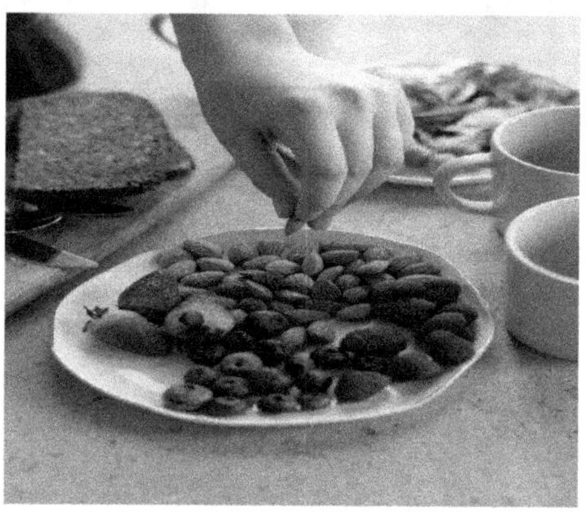

Week 2: Embrace Probiotic Foods

:

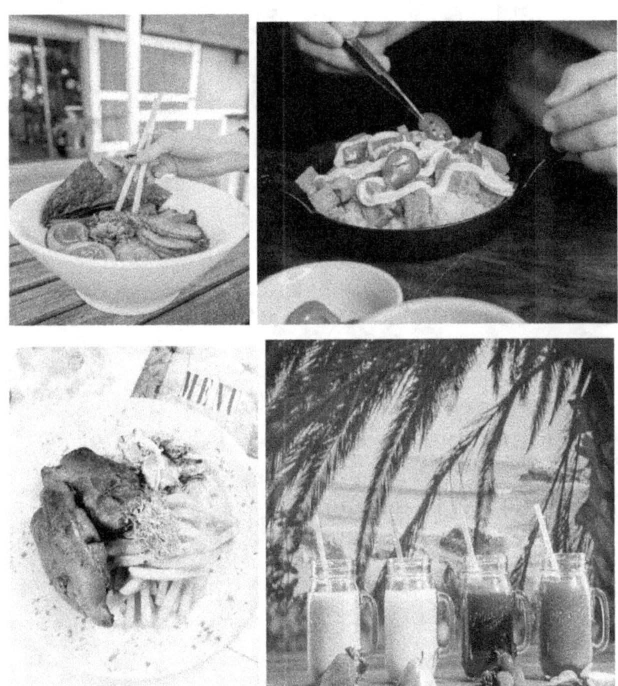

Day 8-14:

- Breakfast:

 - Smoothie with kefir, banana, spinach, and a spoonful of flaxseeds.

Ingredients:

- 1 cup kefir

- 1 ripe banana

- 1 cup fresh spinach leaves

- 1 tablespoon flaxseeds

- 1 tablespoon honey (optional, for sweetness)

- Ice cubes (optional)

Instructions:

1. Place the ripe banana in the blender.

2. Add fresh spinach leaves to the blender for a boost of nutrients.

3. Pour in kefir to the blender for a creamy and probiotic-rich base.

4. Toss in flaxseeds for added fiber and omega-3 fatty acids.

5. Optional: Add a tablespoon of honey if you prefer a sweeter smoothie.

6. Blend until all of the ingredients are smooth and fully incorporated.

7. If desired, add ice cubes to the blender and blend again for a refreshing chill.

8. Pour the smoothie into a glass and garnish with a sprinkle of additional flaxseeds on top.

9. Enjoy this nutritious and delicious kefir banana spinach smoothie as a refreshing breakfast or snack.

This smoothie is not only tasty but also packed with vitamins, minerals, and the goodness of kefir and flaxseeds!

- **Lunch:**

  - Kimchi and tofu stir-fry with brown rice.

Ingredients:

For the Stir-Fry:

- 1 block (14 oz) extra-firm tofu, pressed and cubed

- 1 cup kimchi, chopped

- 1 cup broccoli florets

- 1 carrot, julienned

- 1 red bell pepper, thinly sliced

- 3 green onions, sliced

- 2 tablespoons soy sauce

- 1 tablespoon sesame oil

- 1 tablespoon rice vinegar

- 1 tablespoon gochujang (Korean red pepper paste)

- 2 cloves garlic, minced

- 1 tablespoon grated ginger

- 1 tablespoon vegetable oil for cooking

For Brown Rice:

- 2 cups brown rice

- 4 cups water

- Pinch of salt

Instructions:

For Brown Rice:

1. Rinse the brown rice under cold water until the water runs clear.

2. In a pot, combine the rinsed rice, water, and a pinch of salt.

3. Bring to a boil, then reduce heat, cover, and simmer for about 45-50 minutes or until the rice is tender and water is absorbed.

For Tofu and Kimchi Stir-Fry:

1. In a large wok or skillet, heat vegetable oil over medium-high heat.

2. Add cubed tofu and cook until golden brown on all sides. Remove from the pan and set aside.

3. In the same pan, add more oil if needed and sauté garlic and ginger until fragrant.

4. Add broccoli, carrot, and red bell pepper to the pan. Stir-fry for 3-5 minutes until vegetables are slightly tender.

5. Stir in chopped kimchi and cook for an additional 2-3 minutes.

6. Add the cooked tofu back to the pan.

For the Sauce:

1. In a small bowl, whisk together soy sauce, sesame oil, rice vinegar, and gochujang.

2. Pour the sauce over the tofu and vegetables. Stir well to coat everything evenly.

3. Toss in sliced green onions and continue to stir-fry for an additional 2-3 minutes.

Assemble:

1. Serve the tofu and kimchi stir-fry over a bed of cooked brown rice.

Enjoy this flavorful and nutritious Kimchi and Tofu Stir-Fry with Brown Rice—a perfect combination of savory, spicy, and wholesome goodness!

- **Dinner:**

  - Grilled chicken with sauerkraut, quinoa, and a side of fermented pickles.

Ingredients:

For Grilled Chicken:

- 4 boneless, skinless chicken breasts

- 2 tablespoons olive oil

- 2 teaspoons smoked paprika

- 1 teaspoon garlic powder

- Salt and pepper to taste

For Quinoa:

- 1 cup quinoa, rinsed

- 2 cups chicken or vegetable broth

- 1 tablespoon olive oil

- Salt to taste

For Sauerkraut:

- 2 cups sauerkraut, drained

For Fermented Pickles:

- 1 cup fermented pickles, sliced

Instructions:

For Grilled Chicken:

1. In a bowl, mix olive oil, smoked paprika, garlic powder, salt, and pepper to create a marinade.

2. Coat the chicken breasts with the marinade and let them marinate for at least 30 minutes.

3. Preheat the grill to medium-high heat.

4. Grill the chicken breasts for about 6-8 minutes per side or until fully cooked.

For Quinoa:

1. In a saucepan, combine quinoa, chicken or vegetable broth, olive oil, and a pinch of salt.

2. Bring to a boil, then reduce heat, cover, and simmer for 15-20 minutes or until quinoa is cooked and liquid is absorbed.

For Assembly:

1. Place a portion of cooked quinoa on each plate.

2. Top the quinoa with grilled chicken breasts.

3. Add a generous serving of sauerkraut alongside the chicken.

4. Garnish the plate with slices of fermented pickles.

Serve and Enjoy:

1. Drizzle with additional olive oil or your favorite dressing if desired.

2. Serve immediately and savor the delightful combination of flavors and textures.

This Grilled Chicken with Sauerkraut, Quinoa, and Fermented Pickles is a well-balanced meal with the tanginess of sauerkraut and pickles complementing the smoky grilled chicken and nutty quinoa.

- **Snacks:**

  - Kombucha and a small serving of Greek yogurt with honey.

Ingredients:

For Kombucha:

- 1 bottle of plain or flavored kombucha (store-bought or homemade)

For Greek Yogurt with Honey:

- 1/2 cup Greek yogurt

- 1 tablespoon honey (adjust to taste)

- Optional: Fresh berries or sliced fruits for garnish

Instructions:

For Kombucha:

1. Choose your preferred flavor of kombucha, whether plain or with added fruit flavors.

2. Pour the kombucha into a glass.

3. Optionally, you can add ice cubes for a colder beverage.

For Greek Yogurt with Honey:

1. Spoon Greek yogurt into a small bowl.

2. Drizzle honey over the Greek yogurt.

3. Gently mix the honey into the yogurt, creating a sweet and creamy combination.

4. Optionally, garnish with fresh berries or sliced fruits for added freshness and flavor.

To Serve:

1. Enjoy sipping on the kombucha while savoring spoonfuls of Greek yogurt with honey.

2. Alternate sips and bites for a delightful and refreshing experience.

This simple combination of Kombucha and Greek yogurt with honey offers a balance of tangy, sweet, and creamy flavors, making it a delicious and healthy treat.

Week 3: Boost Fiber Intake

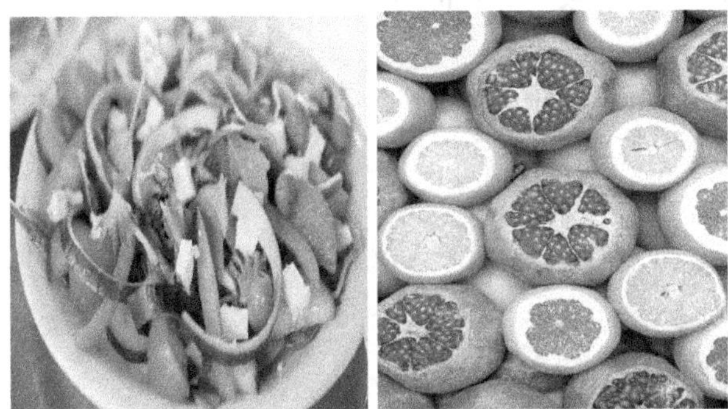

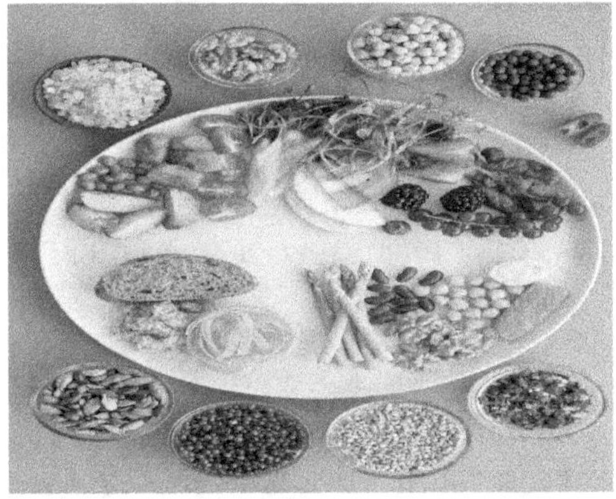

Day 15-21:

- Breakfast:

- Oatmeal topped with sliced strawberries, kiwi, and a sprinkle of pumpkin seeds.

Ingredients:

- 1 cup rolled oats

- 2 cups water or milk

- A pinch of salt

- Sliced strawberries

- Sliced kiwi

- Pumpkin seeds

Instructions:

1. Prepare Oatmeal:

   - Bring water or milk to a boil in a saucepan.

- Add rolled oats and a bit of salt and mix well.

   - Reduce heat and simmer, stirring occasionally, until oats are cooked to your desired consistency.

2. Slice Fruits:

   - While the oatmeal is cooking, slice fresh strawberries and kiwi.

3. Assemble:

   - Once the oatmeal is ready, spoon it into bowls.

   - Top with sliced strawberries and kiwi.

4. Add Pumpkin Seeds:

   - Sprinkle a handful of pumpkin seeds over the fruity oatmeal for a delightful crunch.

5. Optional Sweetener:

   - If desired, drizzle honey or maple syrup on top for added sweetness.

6. Serve:

   - Serve warm and enjoy a delicious and nutritious breakfast packed with flavors and textures.

- **Lunch:**

  - Whole-grain crackers served alongside lentil soup.

Ingredients:

For Whole-Grain Crackers:

- 1 cup whole wheat flour

- 1/2 cup oats

- 1/4 cup flaxseeds, ground

- 1/4 cup sesame seeds

- 1/4 cup olive oil

- 1/2 cup water

- 1/2 teaspoon salt

- 1/2 teaspoon garlic powder (optional)

- 11/2 teaspoon dry herbs (thyme, rosemary)

For the Lentil Soup

:- 1 cup washed dry green or brown lentils

- 1 onion, finely chopped

- 2 carrots, diced

- 2 celery stalks, diced

- 3 cloves garlic, minced

- 1 can diced tomatoes (14 oz)

- 6 cups vegetable broth

- 1 teaspoon cumin

- 1 teaspoon coriander

- 1/2 teaspoon paprika

- Salt and pepper to taste

- Fresh parsley for garnish

Instructions:

1. Prepare Crackers:

   - Preheat oven to 350°F (175°C).

   - In a bowl, mix whole wheat flour, oats,
ground flaxseeds, sesame seeds, olive oil,

water, salt, garlic powder, and dried herbs until a dough forms.

- Roll out the dough on a floured surface and cut into desired cracker shapes.

- Place crackers on a baking sheet and bake for 15-20 minutes or until golden brown.

2. Make Lentil Soup:

- In a large pot, sauté onions, carrots, celery, and garlic until softened.

- Add lentils, diced tomatoes, vegetable broth, cumin, coriander, paprika, salt, and pepper. Bring to a boil, then simmer for about 25-30 minutes until lentils are tender.

3. Serve:

- Ladle the hearty lentil soup into bowls.

- Arrange a handful of whole-grain crackers on the side.

4. Garnish:

- Garnish the lentil soup with fresh parsley.

5. Enjoy:

   - Dip the whole-grain crackers into the flavorful lentil soup for a wholesome and satisfying meal.

This pairing offers a balance of crunchy, whole-grain goodness from the crackers and the heartiness of a well-spiced lentil soup. Perfect for a comforting and nutritious meal!

- **Dinner:**

 - Stir-fried vegetables (bell peppers, broccoli, carrots) with tofu and brown rice.

Ingredients:

For Stir-Fry:

- 1 block extra-firm tofu, pressed and cubed

- 2 cups broccoli florets

- 1 red bell pepper, sliced

- 1 yellow bell pepper, sliced

- 2 carrots, julienned

- 3 cloves garlic, minced

- 1 tablespoon ginger, minced

- 3 tablespoons soy sauce

- 2 tablespoons sesame oil

- 1 tablespoon rice vinegar

- 1 tablespoon maple syrup or honey

- 1 tablespoon cornstarch (optional, for thickening)

- Sesame seeds for garnish

- Green onions, chopped, for garnish

For Brown Rice:

- 1 cup brown rice

- 2 cups water

- Pinch of salt

Instructions:

1. Prepare Brown Rice:

   - Rinse the brown rice under cold water.

   - Combine brown rice, water, and a touch of salt in a pot. Bring to a boil, then lower to a low heat, cover, and leave to cook for 45-50 minutes, or until the rice is cooked.

2. Tofu Preparation: Press the tofu to remove extra water before cutting into cubes.

3. Stir-Fry Tofu: In a large pan or wok, heat sesame oil over medium-high heat.- Stir-fry the tofu cubes until golden brown on all sides.Place aside.

4. Vegetable Stir-Fry: If necessary, add a little extra sesame oil to the same skillet.- Add the minced garlic and ginger and stir until fragrant.- Mix in the broccoli, bell peppers, and carrots. Cook until the veggies are tender-crisp.

5. Combine Tofu and veggies: - Place the tofu back in the skillet with the veggies.

6. Make Sauce:

  - In a small bowl, whisk together soy sauce, rice vinegar, and maple syrup. If you want a thicker sauce, mix in cornstarch with a bit of water and add to the sauce.

7. Combine and Cook:

   - Pour the sauce over the tofu and vegetables. Stir well to coat.

   - Cook for another 2-3 minutes, or until everything is well heated.

8. Serve:

   - Serve the tofu and vegetable stir-fry over brown rice.

   - Garnish with sesame seeds and chopped green onions.

9. Enjoy:

   - Enjoy a delicious and nutritious tofu and vegetable stir-fry with the wholesome goodness of brown rice.

This flavorful stir-fry combines the protein-rich tofu with vibrant vegetables, creating a satisfying meal that's both tasty and wholesome.

- **Snacks:**

  - Fresh vegetable sticks (carrots, cucumber) with hummus and a handful of almonds.

Ingredients:

For Fresh Vegetable Sticks:

- Carrot sticks

- Cucumber sticks

For Hummus:

- 1 can (15 oz) washed and drained chickpeas

- 1/4 cup tahini

- 1/4 cup extra-virgin olive oil

- 2 cloves garlic, minced

- Juice of 1 lemon

- 1/2 teaspoon ground cumin

- Salt and pepper to taste

- 2-3 tablespoons water (for desired consistency)

For Almonds:

- Handful of almonds (raw or roasted)

Instructions:

For Fresh Vegetable Sticks:

1. Wash and peel carrots. Cut them into sticks.

2. Wash and cut cucumber into sticks.

3. Arrange the carrot and cucumber sticks on a serving plate.

For Hummus:

1. Combine chickpeas, tahini, olive oil, minced garlic, lemon juice, ground cumin, salt, and pepper in a food processor.

2. Process the ingredients until smooth, stopping to scrape down the sides as needed.

3. With the food processor running, add water gradually until the hummus reaches your desired creamy consistency.

4. Taste and adjust the seasoning if necessary.

5. Transfer the hummus to a serving bowl.

For Almonds:

1. Place a handful of almonds in a small bowl.

To Serve:

1. Serve the fresh vegetable sticks with the bowl of hummus.

2. Enjoy the vegetable sticks by dipping them into the creamy hummus.

3. Add a handful of almonds on the side for a satisfying and nutritious snack.

This combination makes for a delicious, healthy, and simple snack – perfect for satisfying your hunger with a mix of crunchy vegetables, creamy hummus, and a handful of almonds.

Week 4: Mindful Eating and Hydration

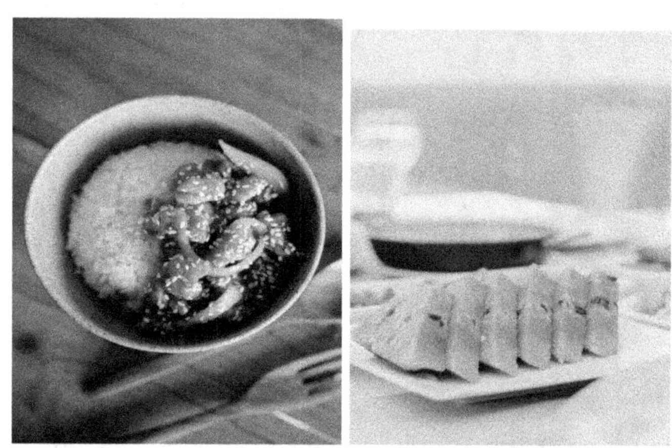

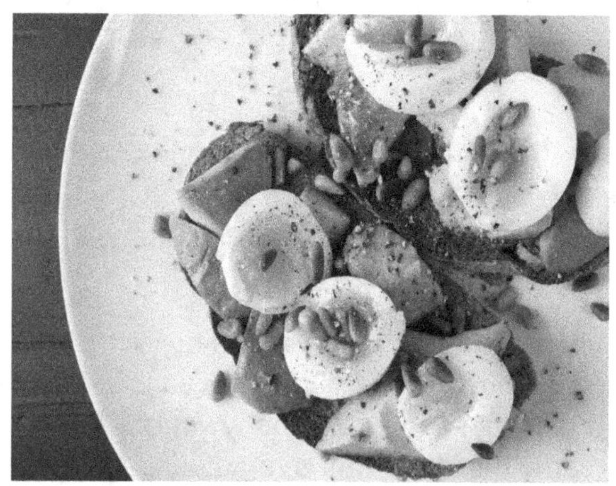

Day 22-28:

- Breakfast:

 - Whole-grain toast with avocado, cherry tomatoes, and poached eggs.

Ingredients:

- 2 slices whole grain bread, toasted

- 1 ripe avocado

- 1 cup cherry tomatoes, halved

- 2 large eggs

- Salt and pepper to taste

- Red pepper flakes (optional)

- Fresh cilantro or parsley for garnish (optional)

- Lemon wedges for serving

Instructions:

1.   - Bring a pot of water to a gentle simmer.

- In the simmering water, create a moderate vortex and delicately slide the eggs into the centre.

- Poach for 3-4 minutes if you want a runny yolk, or longer if you want a harder yolk.Remove with a slotted spoon and drain excess water on a paper towel.

2. - Using a fork, mash the ripe avocado in a bowl.Season with salt and pepper to taste.

3. - Spread the mashed avocado evenly on each slice of toasted whole grain bread.

4. - Arrange halved cherry tomatoes on top of the mashed avocado.

5. - Gently place the poached eggs on the tomatoes.

6. - Season with salt and pepper to taste.

Add red pepper flakes if you like a bit of heat.

7. - Garnish with fresh cilantro or parsley for added freshness.

8. - Serve immediately, with lemon wedges on the side.

9.- Enjoy a delightful and nutritious breakfast with the creamy avocado, juicy tomatoes, and perfectly poached eggs on whole grain toast.

This avocado and poached egg toast is a perfect blend of creamy, savory, and fresh flavors, providing a healthy and satisfying start to your day.

- Lunch:

- Quinoa bowl with roasted Brussels sprouts, butternut squash, and a drizzle of olive oil.

Ingredients:

- 1 cup quinoa, rinsed

- 2 cups Brussels sprouts, trimmed and halved

- 2 cups butternut squash, peeled and diced

- 3 tablespoons olive oil

- 1 teaspoon garlic powder

- 1 teaspoon smoked paprika

- Salt and pepper to taste

- Fresh parsley for garnish (optional)

- Lemon wedges for serving

Instructions:

1. - Preheat the oven to 400°F (200°C).

2. - Combine the quinoa and 2 cups of water in
a medium saucepan.Bring to a boil, then lower
to a low heat, cover, and cook for 15-20
minutes, or until the quinoa is tender and the
water has been absorbed.

3. - On a baking sheet, toss Brussels sprouts
and butternut squash with olive oil, garlic
powder, smoked paprika, salt, and pepper.

   - Spread the vegetables in a single layer and
roast in the preheated oven for 25-30 minutes
or until they are golden and tender.

4. - Fluff the cooked quinoa with a fork and
divide it among serving bowls.

5. - Top the quinoa with the roasted Brussels
sprouts and butternut squash.

6- Drizzle olive oil over the quinoa and roasted
vegetables.

7. - Garnish with fresh parsley for a burst of freshness.

8. - Serve the quinoa bowl warm, with lemon wedges on the side.

9.- Enjoy a delicious and wholesome quinoa bowl featuring the nutty flavor of quinoa, paired with the roasted goodness of Brussels sprouts and butternut squash.

This quinoa bowl is a nutritious and flavorful combination that provides a satisfying mix of textures and tastes, making it a perfect meal for a healthy lunch or dinner.

- Dinner:

 - Baked cod with a side of steamed green beans and a quinoa salad.

Ingredients:

For Baked Cod:

- 4 cod fillets

- 2 tablespoons olive oil

- 1 lemon, juiced

- 2 cloves garlic, minced

- Salt and pepper to taste

- Fresh parsley for garnish

For Steamed Green Beans:

- 2 cups fresh green beans, trimmed

- Salt for boiling

For Quinoa Salad:

- 1 cup quinoa, rinsed

- 2 cups water

- 1 cucumber, diced

- 1 cup cherry tomatoes, halved

- 1/4 cup red onion, finely chopped

- 1/4 cup feta cheese, crumbled

- 2 tablespoons olive oil

- 1 tablespoon balsamic vinegar

- Salt and pepper to taste

- Fresh basil for garnish

Instructions:

1. - Preheat the oven to 400°F (200°C).

2. - In a bowl, mix olive oil, lemon juice, minced garlic, salt, and pepper.

   - Place the cod fillets in a baking dish and brush them with the marinade. Let them marinate for 10-15 minutes.

3. - Bake the cod in the preheated oven for
15-20 minutes or until the fish is opaque and
flakes easily with a fork.

   - Garnish with fresh parsley.

4. - Boil some water in a saucepan or pot

   - Steam green beans for 3-5 minutes until
they are tender-crisp. Drain and set aside.

5. - In a separate pot, combine quinoa and
water. Bring to a boil, then reduce heat, cover,
and simmer for 15-20 minutes or until quinoa is
cooked and water is absorbed.

6. - In a large bowl, combine cooked quinoa,
diced cucumber, cherry tomatoes, red onion,
and crumbled feta cheese.

   - Drizzle with olive oil and balsamic vinegar.
Season with salt and pepper. Toss to combine.

7. - Plate the baked cod alongside a portion of steamed green beans and a generous serving of quinoa salad.

8. - Garnish the quinoa salad with fresh basil.

9- Enjoy a delicious and well-balanced meal with perfectly baked cod, crisp green beans, and a refreshing quinoa salad.

This simple and flavorful dish brings together the mild taste of baked cod, the freshness of steamed green beans, and the vibrant flavors of a quinoa salad for a satisfying and nutritious meal.

- **Snacks:**

  - Hydrating snack: Watermelon cubes. Herbal tea or infused water for variety.

Ingredients:

- Fresh watermelon, cut into bite-sized cubes

For Herbal Tea (Optional):

- Herbal tea bags (mint, chamomile, or your favorite herbal blend)

- Hot water

For Infused Water (Optional):

- Sliced cucumber

- Fresh mint leaves

- Sliced lime or lemon

- Cold water

Instructions:

1. - Cut fresh watermelon into bite-sized cubes. Remove seeds if necessary.

2. Herbal Tea (Optional):

   - Brew your favorite herbal tea according package directions.

- Allow the tea to cool to room temperature or refrigerate it.

3. Infused Water (Optional):

   - Fill a pitcher with cold water.

   - Add sliced cucumber, fresh mint leaves, and sliced lime or lemon to the water.

   - Let the infused water sit in the refrigerator for at least an hour to allow the flavors to meld.

4. - Arrange the watermelon cubes on a plate or in a bowl.

5. - Offer a variety by pairing the watermelon cubes with either the herbal tea or the infused water.

6. - Refresh yourself with the hydrating watermelon cubes and a soothing herbal tea or infused water.

This simple and hydrating snack is not only delicious but also provides a burst of hydration from the watermelon and a refreshing beverage option with herbal tea or infused water.

ADDITIONAL TIPS FOR EACH WEEK

Hydrate: - Consume at least 8 glasses of water every day.For extra hydration, try herbal teas and infused water.

- Mindfulness in Eating: Savour each bite, chew carefully, and eliminate distractions during meals to practise mindful eating.

This vibrant and tasty four-week diet contains a wide spectrum of nutrients and antioxidants from fruits, vegetables, and whole foods, supporting both intestinal health and gastronomic delight.

Adjust portion proportions according to individual requirements and tastes, and feel free to personalise the plan to your liking.Portion sizes should be adjusted based on individual needs and dietary choices.This plan emphasizes a variety of nutrient-dense foods, including those that support gut health. If you have certain dietary limitations or health concerns, you should get personalised guidance from a healthcare expert or a licenced dietitian.

CHAPTER FIVE

Post Four-Week Plan

There are still some other dishes you can try out after the 4-week plan

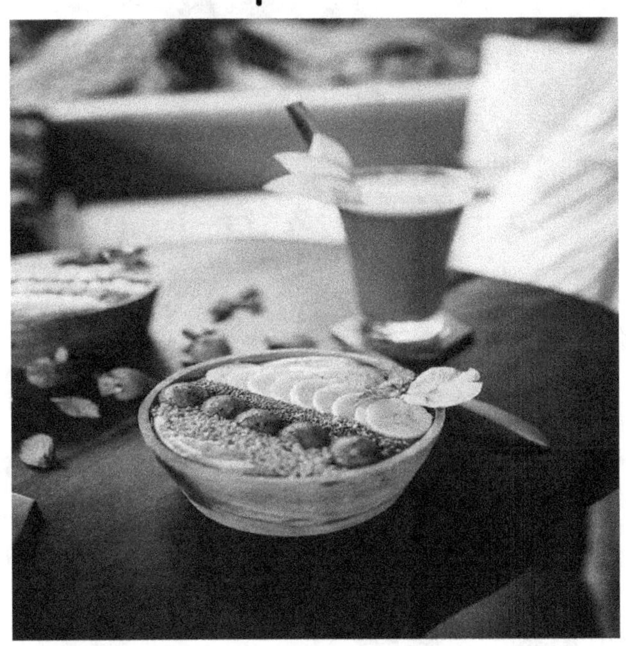

Post Four-Week Recipes

Week 5: Vibrant Gut Rejuvenation

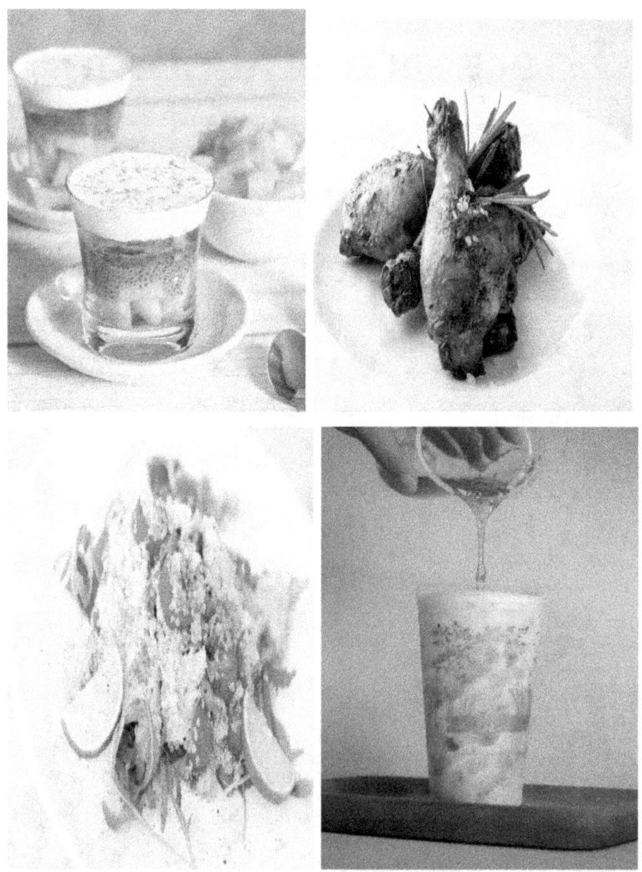

Day 1-7:
- Breakfast:

- Rainbow smoothie bowl with blended berries, mango, spinach, and a sprinkle of seeds.

Ingredients:

For the Smoothie Base:
- 1 cup of frozen berry mixture (raspberries, blueberries, and strawberries)
- 1/2 cup frozen mango chunks
- 1 cup fresh spinach leaves
- 1 ripe banana
- 1/2 cup Greek yogurt
- 1/2 cup almond milk (or any preferred milk)
- 1 tablespoon honey (optional for sweetness)

For Toppings:
- Chia seeds
- Flaxseeds
- Sliced strawberries
- Sliced kiwi
- Fresh blueberries
- Granola

Instructions:

1.- In a blender, combine frozen mixed berries, frozen mango chunks, fresh spinach leaves, ripe banana, Greek yogurt, almond milk, and honey (if using).
   - Blend until smooth and creamy.

2.- Pour the smoothie into a bowl.

3. - Arrange toppings in rows to create a rainbow effect. Place sliced strawberries on one side, followed by sliced kiwi, and then fresh blueberries.

4. - Sprinkle chia seeds and flaxseeds across the smoothie bowl.
   - Add a handful of granola for crunch.

5. - Feel free to get creative with additional toppings like shredded coconut, nuts, or additional fruits.

6. - Present right away and savor with a spoon

7. - Indulge in a vibrant and nutrient-packed rainbow smoothie bowl that combines the goodness of berries, mango, and spinach with a variety of textures and flavors.

This colorful smoothie bowl not only looks beautiful but is also loaded with vitamins, antioxidants, and fiber for a deliciously healthy start to your day.

- Lunch:
- Quinoa-stuffed bell peppers with black beans,
corn, tomatoes, and avocado.

Ingredients:

- 4 1 cup washed quinoa
- 1 big bell pepper, halved and seeds removed
 - 2 cups vegetable broth
 - 1 can (15 oz) washed and drained black beans
- 1 cup corn kernels (fresh or frozen)
- 1 cup cherry tomatoes, diced
- 1 avocado, diced
- 1/2 cup red onion, finely chopped
- 1/4 cup fresh cilantro, chopped
- 1 teaspoon cumin
- 1 teaspoon chili powder
- Salt and pepper to taste
- 1 cup of shredded cheese (optional: Mexican mix
or cheddar)

Instructions:

1.- Preheat the oven to 375°F (190°C).

2. - Combine the quinoa and vegetable broth in a
saucepan.Bring to a boil, then lower to a low heat,
cover, and cook for 15-20 minutes, or until the
quinoa is tender and the water has been absorbed.

3.- Halve the bell peppers lengthwise and remove the seeds and membranes.
- In a baking dish, place the pepper halves.

4.- In a large bowl, combine cooked quinoa, black beans, corn, cherry tomatoes, avocado, red onion, cilantro, cumin, chili powder, salt, and pepper. Mix well.

5. - Fill each bell pepper half with the quinoa mixture, pressing down gently.

6. - If desired, sprinkle shredded cheese on top of each stuffed pepper.

7. - Cover the baking dish with aluminum foil and bake in the preheated oven for 25-30 minutes, or until peppers are tender.

8. - If using cheese, uncover the dish and broil for an additional 2-3 minutes or until the cheese is melted and slightly golden.

9. - Remove from the oven and let it cool slightly before serving.

10.- Enjoy these quinoa-stuffed bell peppers with a delightful mix of flavors and textures from black beans, corn, tomatoes, and avocado.

This healthy and flavorful recipe provides a
satisfying combination of protein, fiber, and
vitamins, making it a delicious and nutritious meal.

- Dinner:
- Grilled chicken or tofu skewers with a side of roasted sweet potatoes and broccoli.

Ingredients:

- 1 lb boneless, skinless chicken breasts or firm tofu, cut into cubes
- 2 tablespoons olive oil
- 2 tablespoons soy sauce
- 1 tablespoon honey or maple syrup
- 1 teaspoon garlic powder
- 1 teaspoon smoked paprika
- Salt and pepper to taste

For the Skewers:

1. In a bowl, mix olive oil, soy sauce, honey (or maple syrup), garlic powder, smoked paprika, salt, and pepper to create a marinade.

2. Thread the chicken/tofu cubes onto skewers and place them in a shallow dish. Pour the marinade over the skewers, making sure each piece is coated. Let it marinate for at least 30 minutes.

3. Preheat your grill or grill pan. Grill the skewers, turning occasionally, until the chicken is cooked through or tofu is nicely grilled.

For the Roasted Sweet Potatoes and Broccoli:

1. Preheat your oven to 400°F (200°C).

2. Peel and dice sweet potatoes into bite-sized cubes. Cut broccoli into florets.

3. Toss sweet potatoes and broccoli with olive oil, salt, and pepper. Spread them on a baking sheet in a single layer.

4. Roast in the preheated oven for about 20-25 minutes or until the sweet potatoes are tender and the broccoli is slightly crispy.

Serve the skewers on a plate alongside the roasted sweet potatoes and broccoli. Enjoy your delicious and nutritious meal!

- Snacks:: Turmeric-Ginger Yogurt Parfait

Ingredients:

For Turmeric-Ginger Yogurt:

- 1 cup Greek yogurt
- 1 teaspoon ground turmeric
- 1 teaspoon fresh ginger, grated
- 1 tablespoon honey or maple syrup
- A pinch of black pepper

For Parfait Assembly:

- Mixed berries (blueberries, raspberries, strawberries)
- Granola (choose a variety with nuts and seeds)
- Chia seeds
- Fresh mint leaves for garnish

Instructions:

1. In a bowl, combine Greek yogurt, ground turmeric, grated ginger, honey (or maple syrup), and a pinch of black pepper. Mix well until the turmeric is evenly distributed.

2. In serving glasses or bowls, start layering the parfait. Begin with a spoonful of the turmeric-ginger yogurt.

3. Add a layer of mixed berries on top of the yogurt.

4. Sprinkle granola on top of the berries.

5. Repeat the layers until the glass or bowl is filled, finishing with a dollop of the turmeric-ginger yogurt on top.

6. Sprinkle chia seeds over the final layer.

7. Garnish with fresh mint leaves for a burst of freshness.

8. Refrigerate for a short time if desired or enjoy immediately.

This Vibrant Gut Rejuvenation Snack, featuring turmeric-ginger yogurt, mixed berries, granola, and chia seeds, is rich in probiotics, antioxidants, and fiber – promoting gut health and providing a burst of flavors and textures.

Week 6: Colors of the Garden

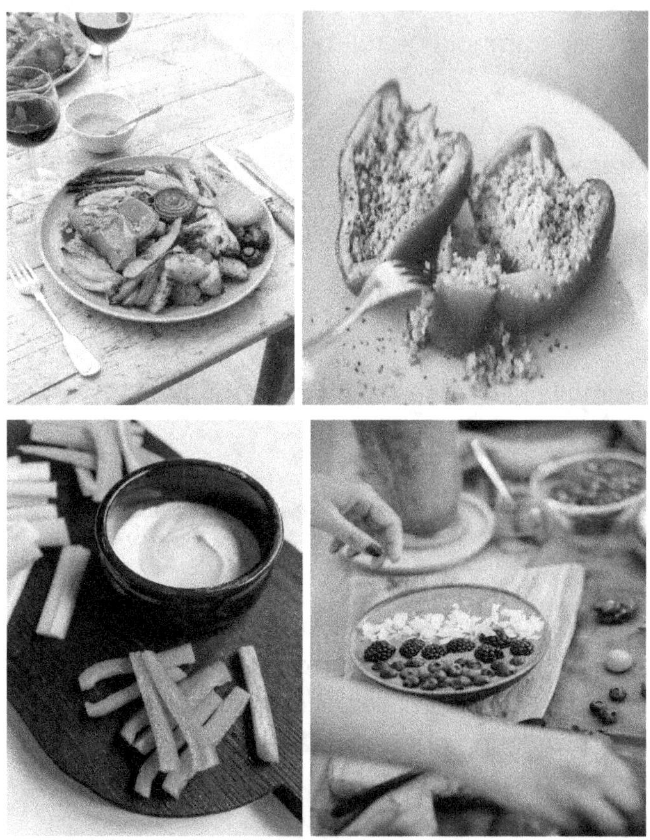

Day 8-14:
-Breakfast:
Mixed berry smoothie bowl topped with granola, chia seeds, and edible flowers.

Ingredients:

- 1 cup mixed berries (strawberries, blueberries, raspberries)
- 1 ripe banana
- 1/2 cup Greek yogurt
- 1/2 cup almond milk (or any milk of your choice)
- 1 tablespoon honey or maple syrup (optional)
- 1/4 cup granola
- 1 tablespoon chia seeds
- Edible flowers for garnish

Instructions:

1. In a blender, combine mixed berries, banana, Greek yogurt, almond milk, and honey (if using). Blend until smooth and creamy.

2. Pour the smoothie into a bowl.

3. Top the smoothie bowl with granola for crunch and chia seeds for added texture and nutrition.

4. Garnish with edible flowers for a touch of beauty and extra freshness.

5. Feel free to get creative with additional toppings like sliced strawberries, coconut flakes, or a drizzle of nut butter.

Note: You can customize the thickness of your smoothie by adjusting the amount of almond milk. Add more for a thinner consistency or less for a thicker bowl.

-Lunch:
Grilled vegetable and hummus wrap with a side of
cucumber and tomato salad.

Ingredients:

For the Wrap:

- Whole-grain wraps or tortillas
- Assorted vegetables (zucchini, bell peppers, red
onion, mushrooms), sliced
- 1 tablespoon olive oil
- Salt and pepper to taste
- Hummus (store-bought or homemade)

For the Cucumber and Tomato Salad:

- 1 cucumber, diced
- 1 cup cherry tomatoes, halved
- 1/4 cup red onion, finely chopped
- Fresh parsley, chopped
- 2 tablespoons olive oil
- 1 tablespoon red wine vinegar
- Salt and pepper to taste

Instructions:

Grilled Vegetable and Hummus Wrap:

1. Heat a grill or grill pan on medium-high.

2. Toss sliced vegetables with olive oil, salt, and pepper. Grill the vegetables until they are tender and slightly charred.

3. Warm the wraps or tortillas according to the package instructions.

4. Spread a generous layer of hummus on each wrap, leaving space around the edges.

5. Place a portion of the grilled vegetables in the center of each wrap.

6. Fold in the sides of the wrap and then roll it up tightly.

Cucumber and Tomato Salad:

1. In a bowl, combine diced cucumber, cherry tomatoes, red onion, and chopped parsley.

2. In a small bowl, whisk together olive oil, red wine vinegar, salt, and pepper. Pour the dressing over the salad and toss gently to combine.

Serve the Grilled Vegetable and Hummus Wrap with a side of Cucumber and Tomato Salad. Enjoy this refreshing and satisfying meal!

-Dinner:
Quinoa-stuffed bell peppers with a medley of colorful bell peppers, black beans, corn, and cilantro.

Ingredients:

- 4 large bell peppers (assorted colors)
- 1 cup quinoa, rinsed
- 2 cups vegetable broth or water
- 1 can (15 oz) drained and rinsed black beans
- 1 cup corn kernels (fresh or frozen)
- 1 cup cherry tomatoes, diced
- 1/2 cup red onion, finely chopped
- 1/2 cup fresh cilantro, chopped
- 1 teaspoon ground cumin
- 1 teaspoon chili powder
- Salt and pepper to taste
- 1 cup shredded cheese (cheddar or Mexican blend), optional

Instructions:

1. Preheat the oven to 375°F (190°C).

2. Remove the tops of the bell peppers and discard the seeds and membranes.

3. In a medium saucepan, bring vegetable broth (or water) to a boil. Add quinoa, reduce heat to low,

cover, and simmer for 15 minutes or until quinoa is cooked and liquid is absorbed.

4. In a large bowl, combine cooked quinoa, black beans, corn, cherry tomatoes, red onion, cilantro, cumin, chili powder, salt, and pepper. Mix well.

5. Stuff each bell pepper with the quinoa mixture, pressing down gently to pack it.

6. If using cheese, sprinkle it over the top of each stuffed pepper.

7. Place the stuffed peppers in a baking dish and cover with aluminum foil.

8. Bake in the preheated oven for 25-30 minutes or until the peppers are tender.

9. Remove the foil and bake for an additional 5-10 minutes to melt the cheese (if added) and lightly brown the tops.

10. Garnish with additional cilantro before serving.

Serve these colorful and flavorful Quinoa-Stuffed Bell Peppers for a wholesome and satisfying meal!

-Snacks:
Crudites platter with rainbow-colored bell pepper strips, cherry tomatoes, and yogurt-based dip.
Ingredients:

For Yogurt-Based Dip:

- 1 cup Greek yogurt
- 1 tablespoon fresh dill, chopped
- 1 tablespoon fresh parsley, chopped
- 1 clove garlic, minced
- 1 tablespoon lemon juice
- Salt and pepper to taste

For Crudites:

- 1 red bell pepper, sliced into strips
- 1 yellow bell pepper, sliced into strips
- 1 orange bell pepper, sliced into strips
- 1 green bell pepper, sliced into strips
- Cherry tomatoes, whole

Instructions:

For Yogurt-Based Dip:

1. In a bowl, combine Greek yogurt, chopped dill, chopped parsley, minced garlic, lemon juice, salt, and pepper.

2. Mix the ingredients thoroughly until well combined.

3. Taste the dip and adjust seasoning if needed. Refrigerate until ready to serve.

For Crudites:

1. Wash and slice the bell peppers into thin strips, creating a rainbow of colors.

2. Arrange the bell pepper strips on a serving platter, creating a visually appealing display.

3. Place cherry tomatoes on the platter alongside the bell pepper strips.

4. Serve the rainbow-colored bell pepper strips and cherry tomatoes with the yogurt-based dip.

5. Enjoy the delicious and healthy crudites platter as a colorful and nutritious snack or appetizer.

This vibrant and flavorful crudites platter is perfect for gatherings or as a refreshing and nutritious snack.

Week 7: Mediterranean Flavors

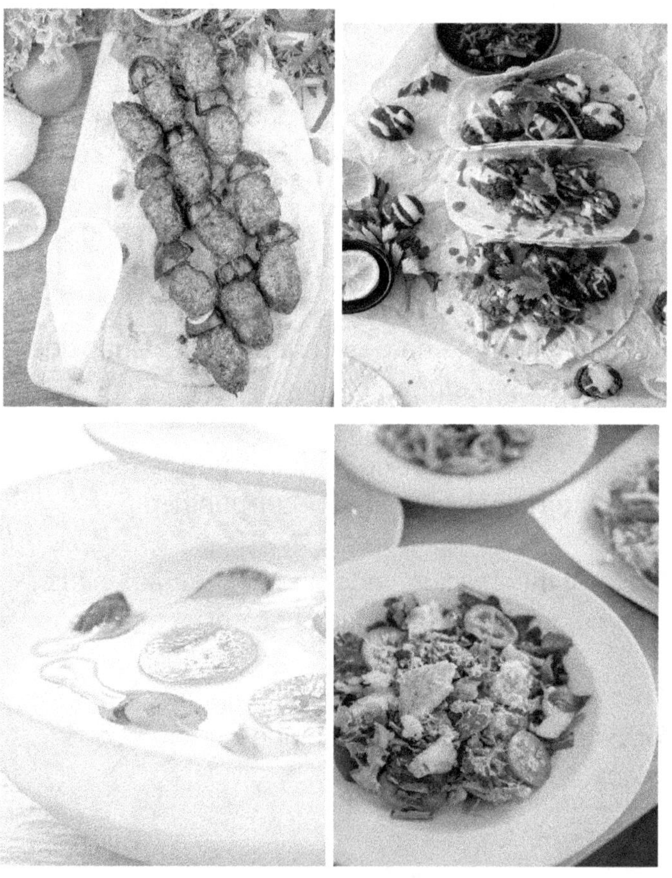

Day 15-21:
- Breakfast:
  - Greek yogurt parfait with layers of mixed berries, granola, and a dollop of honey.

Ingredients:

- 1 cup Greek yogurt
- 1 cup mixed berries (strawberries, blueberries, raspberries)
- 1/2 cup granola
- 2 tablespoons honey

Instructions:

1. In a glass or a bowl, start by layering a spoonful of Greek yogurt at the bottom.

2. Add a layer of mixed berries on top of the yogurt.

3. Sprinkle granola on top of the berries.

4. Drizzle a small amount of honey over the granola.

5. Repeat the layers until you reach the top of the glass or bowl.

6. Finish with a dollop of Greek yogurt, a few berries, and a final drizzle of honey on top.
Grab a long spoon and enjoy

Note: Customize the parfait with your favorite berries, nuts, or seeds for added variety and nutrition.

- Lunch:
  - Chickpea and vegetable Mediterranean salad with feta cheese and a lemon vinaigrette.

Ingredients:
- 1 can (15 oz) of drained and rinsed chickpeas
- 1 cup cherry tomatoes, halved
- 1 cucumber, diced
- 1 bell pepper (any color), diced
- 1/2 red onion, finely chopped
- 1/2 cup Kalamata olives, sliced
- 1/2 cup feta cheese, crumbled
- Fresh parsley, chopped (for garnish)

For Lemon Vinaigrette:
- 1/4 cup extra-virgin olive oil
- 2 tablespoons fresh lemon juice
- 1 teaspoon Dijon mustard
- 1 clove garlic, minced
- Salt and pepper to taste

Instructions:
1. In a large bowl, combine chickpeas, cherry tomatoes, cucumber, bell pepper, red onion, and Kalamata olives.

2. In a separate small bowl, whisk together olive oil, lemon juice, Dijon mustard, minced garlic, salt, and pepper to create the lemon vinaigrette.

3. Pour the vinaigrette over the chickpea and vegetable mixture and toss gently to coat everything evenly.

4. Sprinkle crumbled feta cheese over the salad.

5. To ensure that the flavors fully combine, let the salad marinate in the fridge for at least half an hour.

6. Before serving, garnish with fresh chopped parsley.

Enjoy your refreshing and nutritious Chickpea and Vegetable Mediterranean Salad!

- Dinner:
  - Grilled eggplant and zucchini lasagna with a tomato and basil sauce.

Ingredients:

- 2 large eggplants, sliced lengthwise
- 2 medium zucchinis, sliced lengthwise
- Olive oil for brushing
- Salt and black pepper to taste

For Tomato and Basil Sauce:

- 2 cans (28 oz each) crushed tomatoes
- 3 cloves garlic, minced
- 1/4 cup fresh basil, chopped
- 1 teaspoon dried oregano
- Salt and pepper to taste

For Assembly:

- 1 cup part-skim ricotta cheese
- 1 cup shredded mozzarella cheese
- 1/2 cup grated Parmesan cheese
- Fresh basil leaves for garnish

Instructions:

1. Preheat the grill or grill pan. Brush eggplant and zucchini slices with olive oil and season with salt and pepper.

2. Grill the eggplant and zucchini slices until tender and grill marks appear, about 3-4 minutes per side. Set aside.

3. In a saucepan, combine crushed tomatoes, minced garlic, chopped basil, dried oregano, salt, and pepper. Simmer the sauce over medium heat for 15-20 minutes, allowing the flavors to meld.

4. Preheat the oven to 375°F (190°C).

5. In a baking dish, spread a thin layer of tomato and basil sauce. Layer grilled eggplant and zucchini slices over the sauce.

6. Spread half of the ricotta cheese over the grilled vegetables, followed by a portion of the mozzarella and Parmesan cheeses.

7. Repeat the layers, finishing with a layer of tomato and basil sauce and a generous sprinkle of mozzarella and Parmesan.

8. Bake for 25 to 30 minutes, or until the cheese is bubbling and melted, in a preheated oven.

9. Before serving, let the lasagna sit for a few minutes.

- Snacks:
  - Hummus with multicolored bell pepper strips.
Ingredients:

For Hummus:

- 1 can (15 oz) of drained and rinsed chickpeas
- 1/4 cup tahini
- 1/4 cup extra-virgin olive oil
- 2 cloves garlic, minced
- Juice of 1 lemon
- 1/2 teaspoon ground cumin
- Salt and pepper to taste
- 2-3 tablespoons water (for desired consistency)

For Multicolored Bell Pepper Strips:

- 1 red bell pepper, sliced into strips
- 1 yellow bell pepper, sliced into strips
- 1 orange bell pepper, sliced into strips
- 1 green bell pepper, sliced into strips

Instructions:

For Hummus:

1. Place the chickpeas, ground cumin, lemon juice, olive oil, chopped garlic, tahini, salt, and pepper in a food processor.

2. Process the ingredients until smooth, stopping to scrape down the sides as needed.

3. With the food processor running, add water gradually until the hummus reaches your desired creamy consistency.

4. Taste and adjust the seasoning if necessary.

For Multicolored Bell Pepper Strips:

1. Wash and slice the bell peppers into thin strips.

2. Arrange the multicolored bell pepper strips on a serving platter.

Serve the hummus alongside the multicolored bell pepper strips for a colorful, delicious, and healthy snack or appetizer. Enjoy!

Week 8: Fusion Fiesta

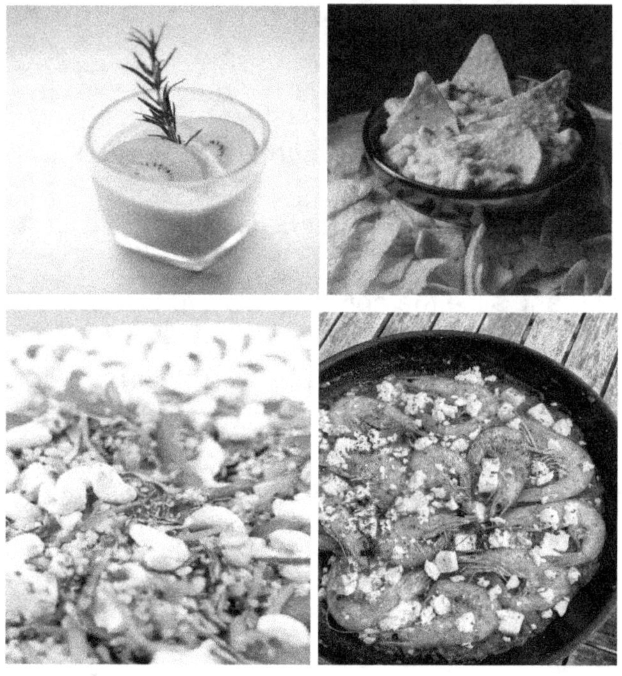

Day 22-28:
- Breakfast:
 - Tropical fruit smoothie with pineapple, kiwi, and mango.

Ingredients:

- 1 cup fresh pineapple, diced
- 1 ripe mango, peeled and diced
- 2 kiwi fruits, peeled and sliced
- 1 banana, peeled

- 1/2 cup Greek yogurt
- 1 cup coconut water or almond milk
- Ice cubes (optional)
- Honey or agave syrup (optional, for sweetness)

Instructions:

1. Place diced pineapple, mango, kiwi, banana, and Greek yogurt in a blender.

2. Pour in coconut water or almond milk.

3. Optional: Add ice cubes for a colder and thicker consistency.

4. Blend until all the ingredients are smooth and creamy.

5. Taste the smoothie and add honey or agave syrup if you desire additional sweetness.

6. Pour the tropical fruit smoothie into glasses and serve immediately.

Enjoy your refreshing and nutritious Tropical Fruit Smoothie with Pineapple, Kiwi, and Mango!

- Lunch:
  - Shrimp or tofu stir-fry with a variety of colorful vegetables and sesame ginger sauce.
Ingredients:

- 1 pound shrimp, peeled and deveined (or firm tofu, cubed for a vegetarian option)
- 2 cups broccoli florets
- 1 thinly sliced bell pepper, (use a mix of colors for vibrancy)
- 1 carrot, julienned
- 1 cup snap peas, ends trimmed
- 3 green onions, sliced
- 3 cloves garlic, minced
- 1 tablespoon fresh ginger, grated
- 2 tablespoons sesame oil, divided
- 1/4 cup low-sodium soy sauce
- 2 tablespoons rice vinegar
- 1 tablespoon honey or maple syrup
- 1 tablespoon cornstarch (optional, for thickening)
- Sesame seeds and chopped cilantro for garnish
- Cooked brown rice or quinoa for serving

Instructions:

1. In a small bowl, whisk together soy sauce, rice vinegar, honey (or maple syrup), and cornstarch (if using). Set aside.

2. In a large skillet or wok, heat 1 tablespoon of sesame oil over medium-high heat.

3. Add shrimp or tofu to the skillet and cook until shrimp turn pink or tofu becomes golden brown. Remove from the skillet and set aside.

4. In the same skillet, add the remaining tablespoon of sesame oil. Stir in minced garlic and grated ginger, sautéing for about 30 seconds until fragrant.

5. Add broccoli, bell pepper, carrot, and snap peas to the skillet. Stir-fry the vegetables for 3-5 minutes or until they are tender-crisp.

6. Return the cooked shrimp or tofu to the skillet, along with the sliced green onions.

7. Pour the sesame ginger sauce over the stir-fry and toss everything together until well-coated and heated through.

8. Serve the shrimp or tofu stir-fry over cooked brown rice or quinoa.

9. Garnish with sesame seeds and chopped cilantro.

Enjoy your delicious and healthy Shrimp or Tofu Stir-Fry with Colorful Vegetables and Sesame Ginger Sauce!

- Dinner:
  - Quinoa paella with a medley of bell peppers, tomatoes, peas, and saffron.
Ingredients:

- 1 cup quinoa, rinsed and drained
- 2 cups vegetable broth
- 1/4 teaspoon saffron threads
- 2 tablespoons olive oil
- 1 onion, finely chopped
- 3 cloves garlic, minced
- 1 red bell pepper, diced
- 1 yellow bell pepper, diced
- 1 orange bell pepper, diced
- 1 cup cherry tomatoes, halved
- 1 cup frozen peas, thawed
- 1 teaspoon smoked paprika
- 1 teaspoon dried oregano
- Salt and black pepper to taste
- Lemon wedges for serving
- Fresh parsley, chopped (for garnish)

Instructions:

1. In a small bowl, combine saffron threads with 2 tablespoons of warm water. Let it steep.

2. In a medium saucepan, bring vegetable broth to a boil. After adding the quinoa, lower the heat to simmer, cover, and let the quinoa cook for 15 to 20 minutes, or until the liquid has been absorbed.

3. Heat the olive oil in a big pan over medium heat.

4. Add diced bell peppers to the skillet and cook for 3-4 minutes until they begin to soften.

5. Stir in cherry tomatoes, thawed peas, smoked paprika, dried oregano, saffron with its liquid, salt, and black pepper. Cook for an additional 3-4 minutes until tomatoes are slightly softened.

6. Add the cooked quinoa to the skillet, tossing everything together until well combined and heated through.

7. Adjust seasoning if needed. Serve the quinoa paella with lemon wedges on the side.

8. Garnish with chopped fresh parsley before serving.

Enjoy your delicious and healthy Quinoa Paella with a Medley of Bell Peppers, Tomatoes, Peas, and Saffron!

- Snacks:
  - Guacamole with whole-grain tortilla chips.

Ingredients:

For Guacamole:
- 3 ripe avocados, peeled and pitted
- 1 medium tomato, diced
- 1/4 cup red onion, finely chopped
- 1 clove garlic, minced
- 1 jalapeño, seeded and finely chopped (optional for heat)
- Juice of 1 lime
- Salt and pepper to taste
- Fresh cilantro, chopped (optional for garnish)

For Whole-Grain Tortilla Chips:
- Whole-grain tortillas
- Olive oil spray
- Sea salt

Instructions:

For Guacamole:

1. In a bowl, mash the ripe avocados with a fork or potato masher until smooth, leaving some chunks for texture.

2. Add diced tomato, chopped red onion, minced garlic, jalapeño (if using), and lime juice to the mashed avocados. Mix well.

3. To taste, add salt and pepper to the guacamole. Adjust lime juice or salt as needed.

4. Optional: Garnish with chopped fresh cilantro.

For Whole-Grain Tortilla Chips:

1. Preheat the oven to 350°F (175°C).

2. Cut whole-grain tortillas into triangles or desired shapes.

3. Arrange the tortilla pieces on a baking sheet in a single layer.

4. Lightly spray the tortillas with olive oil and sprinkle sea salt over them.

5. Bake in the preheated oven for 10-12 minutes or until the chips are golden and crisp.

6. Allow the tortilla chips to cool before serving.

Serve the fresh guacamole with the whole-grain tortilla chips, and enjoy your delicious and healthy snack!

Additional Tips:
- Experiment with herbs and spices to add flavor without excessive salt or sugar.
- Include fermented foods like kimchi or sauerkraut for an extra probiotic boost.
- Drink herbal teas or infusions to stay hydrated.
- Try different cooking methods: grilling, roasting, steaming, and sautéing to enhance flavors and textures.

Adjust portion sizes based on individual needs and dietary preferences. This plan emphasizes a variety of nutrient-dense foods, including those that support gut health. Seeking individualized counsel from a qualified dietician or healthcare expert is advised if you have any health issues or special dietary limitations.

Conclusion

In conclusion, this Secret of Gut Health Cookbook unveils a culinary journey that transcends mere recipes; it's a profound exploration of the symbiotic relationship between nourishment and well-being.

By embracing the art of mindful eating and harnessing the transformative power of gut-friendly ingredients, this cookbook not only enriches our palates but also fosters a harmonious connection between our bodies and the food we consume. Through an array of delectable dishes and insightful nutritional wisdom, it empowers readers to embark on a transformative voyage towards digestive vitality.

 As you savor the flavors and embrace the culinary revelations within these pages, you're not just cooking; you're cultivating a sanctuary of well-being within, where the secrets to gut health unfolds in every delicious bite.
Cheers to a healthier, more vibrant you!

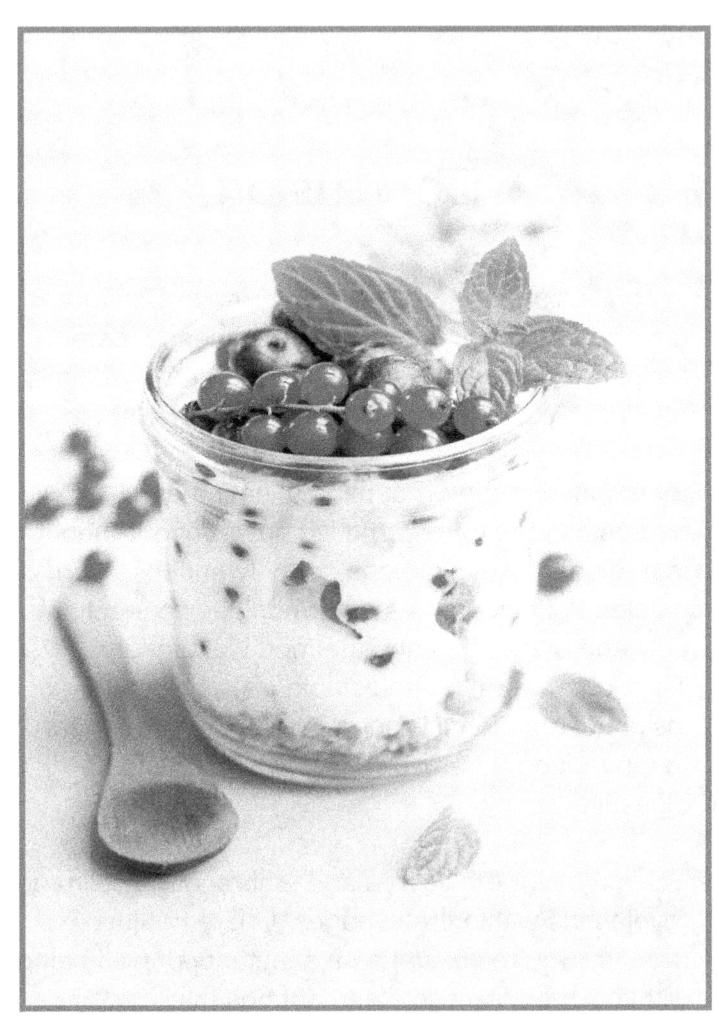